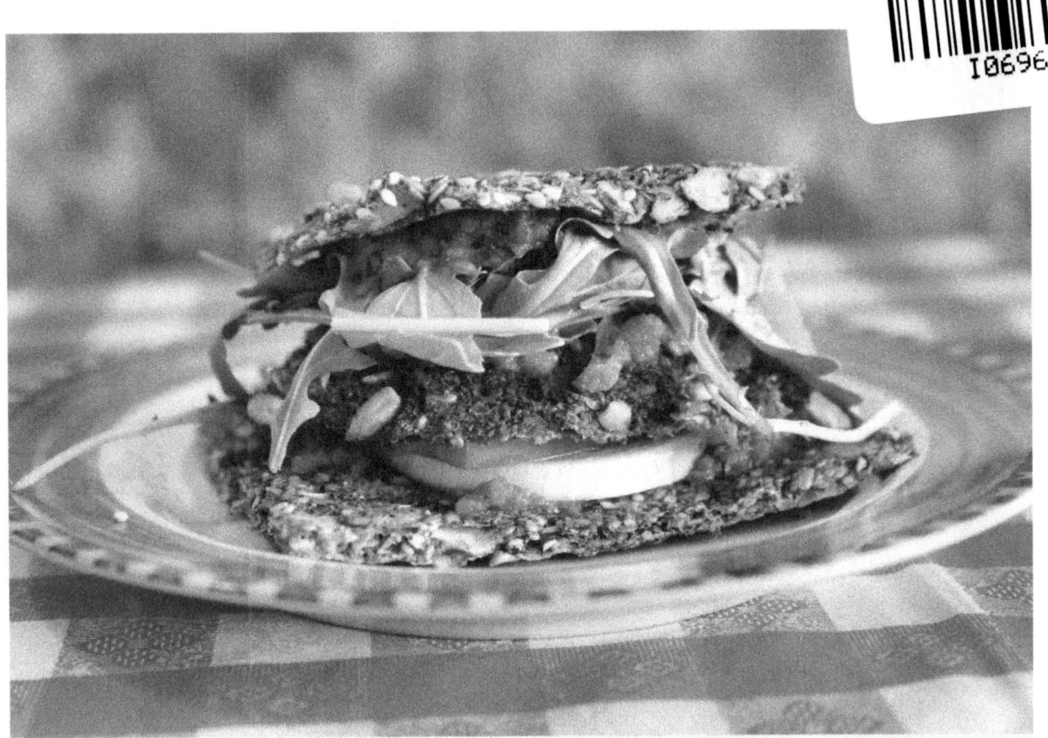

UNCOOKED

A raw foods cookbook for the
adventurous eater.....

By William Davenport

Raw food is the best way to have the cleanest energy. We take so much care about what kind of fuel we put in our car, what kind of oil. We care about that sometimes more than the fuel that we're looking at putting in our bodies. It's cleaner burning fuel. - Woody Harrelson

Prologue: The Benefits of Raw Food Diets

In recent years, the popularity of raw food diets has soared among health-conscious individuals seeking optimal well-being and a vibrant lifestyle. Raw food diets encompass various approaches, including raw vegan, raw paleo, raw fruitarian, raw juice, raw vegetarian, raw dairy-free, raw gluten-free, raw nut-based, raw alkaline, and raw superfood diets. Regardless of the specific approach, these diets share one common principle: consuming uncooked, unprocessed, and nutrient-rich foods.

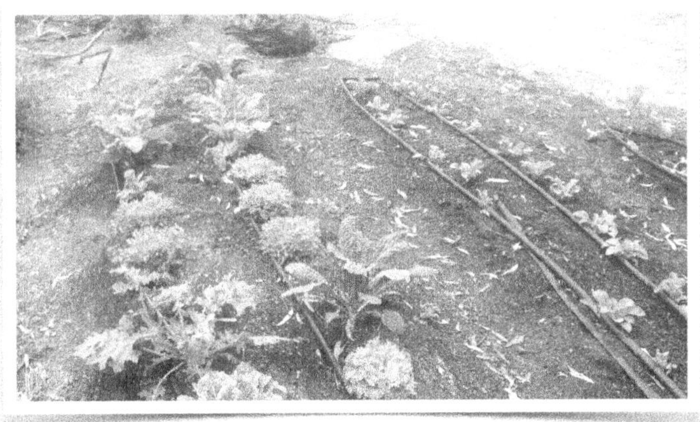

William's Garden

Chapter 1: Introduction to Raw Food Diet

One of the key benefits of raw food diets is the preservation of vital nutrients. Raw fruits, vegetables, nuts, and seeds are packed with essential vitamins, minerals, enzymes, and antioxidants that can be partially destroyed during cooking. By consuming these foods in their natural, uncooked state, individuals can maximize their nutrient intake, leading to improved energy levels, enhanced immune function, and reduced risk of chronic diseases. Raw food diets are also known for their ability to support weight loss and weight management. Raw foods are generally low in calories and high in fiber, making them ideal for those seeking to shed excess pounds. Additionally, the high water content in raw fruits and vegetables helps to create a feeling of fullness, preventing overeating and promoting satiety. Raw foods are rich in enzymes that aid in the digestive process, reducing the burden on the body's enzymatic systems. This can lead to better nutrient absorption, reduced bloating, and improved bowel regularity.

Another advantage of adopting a raw food diet is its potential to boost mental clarity and emotional well-being. The abundance of nutrients found in raw foods supports brain health and cognitive function, leading to increased focus, concentration, and overall mental sharpness. Additionally, raw food diets are often associated with reduced inflammation, which can positively impact mood and emotional stability.

A raw food diets are environmentally friendly and sustainable. By focusing on plant-based foods and minimizing reliance on processed and packaged products, individuals can reduce their carbon footprint and contribute to a more sustainable food system. Raw food diets also promote ethical considerations by advocating for the compassionate treatment of animals and the avoidance of animal products.

Raw foods offer a multitude of benefits to health-conscious individuals seeking to optimize their well-being. From improved nutrient intake and weight management to enhanced digestion and mental clarity, these diets have the potential to revolutionize one's health and vitality. Whether you choose to follow a raw vegan, raw paleo, or any other raw food approach, embracing the power of raw foods can lead to a truly transformative wellness journey.

In recent years, there has been a significant surge in the popularity of raw food diets among health-conscious individuals. This subchapter aims to delve into the intricacies of the raw food revolution and provide a comprehensive guide for those interested in adopting this lifestyle. Whether you follow a raw vegan, raw paleo, raw fruitarian, raw juice, raw vegetarian, raw dairy-free, raw gluten-free, raw nut-based, raw alkaline, or raw superfood diet, this chapter will equip you with the necessary knowledge to embark on your raw food journey.

The raw food revolution is founded on the principle of consuming unprocessed, uncooked, and organic foods. This lifestyle choice is rooted in the belief that cooking food above a certain temperature destroys essential enzymes, vitamins, and minerals, thereby diminishing its nutritional value. By consuming raw foods, individuals aim to maximize the intake of nutrients and enhance overall health and well-being.

One of the key benefits of a raw food diet is its ability to promote weight loss and maintain a healthy body weight. Raw foods are generally low in calories and high in fiber, which helps to keep you feeling satiated for longer periods. Moreover, the abundance of nutrients in raw foods ensures that your body receives the necessary fuel to function optimally while shedding excess pounds.

The raw food revolution offers numerous health benefits. Raw foods are rich in antioxidants, which help to combat free radicals and reduce the risk of chronic diseases such as heart disease and certain types of cancer. Furthermore, raw food diets have been linked to improved digestion, increased energy levels, clearer skin, and enhanced mental clarity.

However, it is essential to approach the raw food revolution with caution and ensure that your dietary needs are met adequately. By understanding the raw food revolution, you can embark on a journey towards optimal health and well-being. Whether you choose to follow a raw vegan, raw paleo, raw fruitarian, raw juice, raw vegetarian, raw dairy-free, raw gluten-free, raw nut-based, raw alkaline, or raw superfood diet,

Transitioning to a Raw Food Diet

If you are a health-conscious individual looking to improve your overall well-being and embrace a lifestyle that promotes optimal health, transitioning to a raw food diet might be the perfect choice for you. In this subchapter, we will explore the various aspects of transitioning to a raw food diet and how it can benefit different niches such as the raw vegan diet, raw paleo diet, raw fruitarian diet, raw juice diet, raw vegetarian diet, raw dairy-free diet, raw gluten-free diet, raw nut-based diet, raw alkaline diet, and raw superfood diet.

Transitioning to a raw food diet involves incorporating predominantly uncooked and unprocessed foods into your daily meals. This includes fruits, vegetables, nuts, seeds, and sprouted grains. It eliminates the consumption of cooked, processed, and refined foods that often lack essential nutrients and enzymes vital for optimal health.

For those on a raw vegan diet, transitioning means embracing a plant-based lifestyle that excludes all animal products. This diet is abundant in fruits, vegetables, nuts, and seeds, providing ample amounts of vitamins, minerals, and antioxidants.

Raw paleo enthusiasts focus on consuming uncooked and unprocessed foods that mimic what our early ancestors ate. This includes raw meats, fish, eggs, fruits, vegetables, nuts, and seeds. It aims to provide a nutrient-dense diet while avoiding modern processed foods.

If you are considering a raw fruitarian diet, you will primarily consume fresh, raw fruits. This niche diet is rich in vitamins, minerals, and antioxidants, promoting detoxification and weight loss.

The raw juice diet involves consuming freshly squeezed juices from fruits and vegetables. This diet is highly detoxifying and provides a concentrated source of nutrients in an easily digestible form.

For those following a raw vegetarian diet, transitioning involves embracing a plant-based lifestyle that includes raw fruits, vegetables, nuts, and seeds. It excludes all animal products, including meat, fish, eggs, and dairy.

Individuals with dietary restrictions can also benefit from transitioning to a raw food diet. A raw dairy-free diet eliminates all dairy products, while a raw gluten-free diet avoids gluten-containing grains. A raw nut-based diet focuses on incorporating a variety of nuts and seeds into meals.

Moreover, transitioning to a raw alkaline diet can help balance the body's pH levels and promote overall health. This diet includes alkaline-forming foods such as leafy greens, sprouts, and non-sweet fruits.

Lastly, the raw superfood diet incorporates nutrient-dense foods like spirulina, chlorella, and wheatgrass, providing an extra boost of vitamins and minerals.

Transitioning to a raw food diet requires careful planning, education, and experimentation with different recipes and food combinations. It is essential to ensure you meet your nutritional needs and maintain a balanced diet. Gradual changes and seeking guidance from a healthcare professional or a qualified nutritionist can make the transition smoother and more sustainable.

Embracing a raw food diet offers numerous benefits, including increased energy levels, improved digestion, weight loss, enhanced mental clarity, and a strengthened immune system. By transitioning to a raw food diet, you are embarking on a journey towards optimal health and well-being.

Chapter 2: The Raw Food Basics

What is a Raw Food Diet?

In today's world, where processed and artificial foods dominate the grocery store shelves, it's no wonder that more and more health-conscious individuals are turning to a raw food diet. But what exactly does it mean to follow a raw food diet? Let's dive into the world of raw food and explore its various forms and benefits.

Simply put, a raw food diet is one that primarily consists of uncooked, unprocessed, and organic foods. This way of eating is based on the belief that cooking destroys the natural enzymes and nutrients present in food, leading to a loss of vital health benefits. By consuming food in its raw and natural state, proponents of this diet claim to experience increased energy levels, improved digestion, weight loss, and a reduced risk of chronic diseases.

There are several variations of the raw food diet, each with its own unique approach and focus. Let's take a closer look at some popular subcategories:

1. Raw Vegan Diet: This diet excludes all animal products, including meat, dairy, and eggs. It emphasizes consuming a variety of fruits, vegetables, nuts, and seeds.

2. Raw Paleo Diet: This diet combines raw foods with the principles of the paleo diet, which advocates for consuming foods similar to those available to our ancestors. It includes raw meat, fish, fruits, vegetables, nuts, and seeds.

3. Raw Fruitarian Diet: This diet primarily consists of raw fruits, nuts, and seeds. It emphasizes eating fruits that have fallen naturally from trees or plants.

4. Raw Juice Diet: This diet involves consuming freshly squeezed juices from fruits and vegetables. It is believed to provide a concentrated dose of nutrients and enzymes.

5. Raw Vegetarian Diet: This diet excludes meat but includes dairy products and eggs. It focuses on consuming raw fruits, vegetables, nuts, and seeds.

6. Raw Dairy-Free Diet: This diet excludes all dairy products and instead focuses on raw fruits, vegetables, nuts, and seeds.

7. Raw Gluten-Free Diet: This diet avoids gluten-containing grains like wheat, barley, and rye. It includes raw fruits, vegetables, nuts, and seeds.

8. Raw Nut-Based Diet: This diet includes a variety of raw nuts and seeds as the primary source of calories and nutrients.

9. Raw Alkaline Diet: This diet emphasizes consuming alkaline-forming foods such as leafy greens, sprouts, and raw fruits and vegetables to maintain the body's pH balance.

10. Raw Superfood Diet: This diet incorporates nutrient-dense superfoods like spirulina, chlorella, and maca powder into a primarily raw food diet.

No matter which variation of the raw food diet you choose, it's important to ensure that you are meeting your nutritional needs. It may be necessary to supplement certain nutrients like vitamin B12, iron, and omega-3 fatty acids, which are typically found in animal products.

Before embarking on any new diet, it's always advisable to consult with a healthcare professional or registered dietitian to ensure that it aligns with your specific health needs and goals.

A raw food diet offers a unique and natural approach to nourishing your body. By embracing the power of whole, unprocessed foods, you can experience a multitude of health benefits and embark on a journey towards a healthier, more vibrant life.

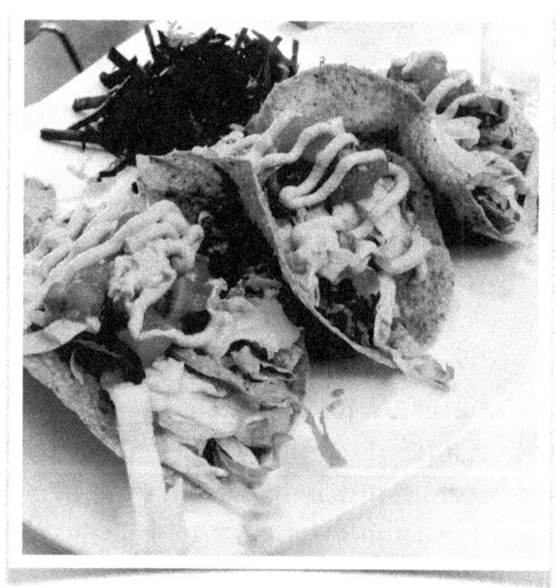

Raw Vegan Tacos

Chapter 3: Raw Food Principles and Philosophy

In this chapter, we will delve into the fundamental principles and philosophy behind the raw food movement. Whether you follow a raw food diet, raw vegan diet, raw paleo diet, raw fruitarian diet, raw juice diet, raw vegetarian diet, raw dairy-free diet, raw gluten-free diet, raw nut-based diet, raw alkaline diet, or raw superfood diet, this chapter will provide you with valuable insights and knowledge.

At its core, the raw food movement promotes the consumption of uncooked, unprocessed, and organic foods in their natural state. The philosophy behind this lifestyle is rooted in the belief that cooking and processing foods can deplete vital nutrients and enzymes, leading to decreased health and vitality. By consuming raw foods, individuals aim to maximize nutrient intake and support optimal health.

One of the key principles of the raw food philosophy is the belief in the healing power of nature. Raw food enthusiasts recognize that fruits, vegetables, nuts, and seeds are abundant sources of vitamins, minerals, antioxidants, and enzymes that can nourish and rejuvenate the body. By embracing raw foods, individuals can tap into the incredible healing potential that nature provides.

Another principle of the raw food movement is the emphasis on sustainability and ethical practices. Health-conscious individuals understand the importance of choosing organic and locally sourced

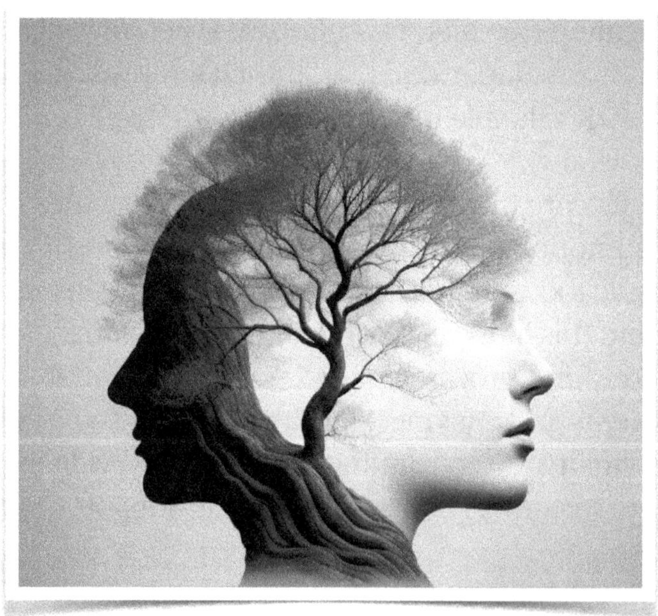

produce to minimize exposure to harmful pesticides and support sustainable farming practices. By opting for raw, plant-based foods, individuals can contribute to a more environmentally friendly and compassionate lifestyle.

The raw food philosophy emphasizes the importance of listening to one's body and intuitive eating. Raw food enthusiasts believe in connecting with their bodies and honoring their unique nutritional needs. By tuning into their body's signals, individuals can make informed choices about their diet and lifestyle, promoting overall well-being.

The principles and philosophy behind the raw food movement offer health-conscious individuals a comprehensive guide to optimal nutrition and vitality. By embracing raw foods, individuals can nourish their bodies with nutrient-dense, unprocessed, and organic foods while supporting sustainable farming practices. The raw food philosophy encourages individuals to listen to their bodies and make intuitive choices about their diet, promoting a harmonious connection between body, mind, and nature.

Chapter 4: The Importance of Enzymes in Raw Foods

In the world of health-conscious individuals, there is a growing movement towards raw food diets. These diets encompass various niches such as raw vegan, raw paleo, raw fruitarian, raw juice, raw vegetarian, raw dairy-free, raw gluten-free, raw nut-based, raw alkaline, and raw superfood diets. While each of these diets has its own unique principles, they all share one common belief - the importance of enzymes in raw foods.

Enzymes are naturally occurring substances that play a vital role in our bodies. They act as catalysts for various chemical reactions, including the digestion and absorption of nutrients. Unfortunately, many of the enzymes present in our food are destroyed through cooking and processing. This is where raw foods come into the picture.

Raw foods, by definition, are uncooked and unprocessed. This means that they retain their natural enzymes, which are crucial for optimal digestion and overall health. When we consume raw foods, these enzymes work harmoniously with our own digestive enzymes to break down food and extract nutrients more efficiently. As a result, our bodies are better able to absorb vitamins, minerals, and other essential compounds.

The benefits of enzymes in raw foods extend beyond digestion. Enzymes also play a role in reducing inflammation, promoting detoxification, and boosting our immune system. They have been linked to improved energy levels, enhanced mental clarity, and even weight loss. In essence, enzymes are the key to unlocking the full potential of raw foods.

For those following a raw food diet, incorporating a variety of enzyme-rich foods is essential. Fruits, vegetables, sprouts, nuts, and seeds are all excellent sources of enzymes. Fermented foods like sauerkraut and kimchi also contain beneficial enzymes. Additionally, certain superfoods such as spirulina, chlorella, and wheatgrass are known for their enzyme content.

It is important to note that while raw foods are a great source of enzymes, our bodies also produce their own digestive enzymes. However, as we age, our enzyme production decreases, making it even more crucial to consume enzyme-rich foods.

Enzymes are a fundamental component of raw foods. They facilitate digestion, improve nutrient absorption, and contribute to overall health and vitality. Whether you follow a raw vegan, raw paleo, raw fruitarian, or any other raw food diet, embracing the importance of enzymes will undoubtedly enhance your well-being. So, go ahead and explore the wonderful world of raw foods, and let the enzymes work their magic on your health.

Essential Nutrients in Raw Foods

In the quest for optimal health, many health-conscious individuals have turned to raw food diets as a means to nourish their bodies with the purest, most natural form of sustenance. Whether you follow a raw vegan, raw paleo, raw fruitarian, raw juice, raw vegetarian, raw dairy-free, raw gluten-free, raw nut-based, raw alkaline, or raw superfood diet, understanding the essential nutrients found in raw foods is crucial for achieving and maintaining optimal well-being.

Raw foods, by definition, are uncooked and unprocessed, allowing them to retain their maximum nutritional value. These nutrient-dense foods are rich in vitamins, minerals, antioxidants, enzymes, and phytonutrients that play vital roles in supporting various bodily functions and promoting overall health.

One of the key benefits of a raw food diet is the abundance of vitamins and minerals found in raw fruits, vegetables, nuts, and seeds. These essential nutrients are vital for maintaining a strong immune system, supporting healthy bones and teeth, and promoting optimal brain function. Raw foods are particularly rich in vitamin C, vitamin A, vitamin K, potassium, magnesium, and folate, which are essential for energy production, skin health, and cardiovascular health.

In addition to vitamins and minerals, raw foods are also a great source of antioxidants. Antioxidants help protect the body from harmful free radicals that can damage cells and contribute to chronic diseases. Raw fruits and vegetables, such as berries, leafy greens, and citrus fruits, are particularly high in antioxidants, including vitamin C, vitamin E, and beta-carotene.

Enzymes are another vital component of raw foods. Enzymes are responsible for facilitating the body's various biochemical reactions, including digestion and nutrient absorption. Raw foods contain naturally occurring enzymes that can support optimal digestion and nutrient assimilation, leading to improved overall digestion and increased nutrient absorption.

Raw foods are an excellent source of fiber, which is essential for maintaining a healthy digestive system, regulating blood sugar levels, and promoting satiety. Raw fruits, vegetables, nuts, and seeds are packed with dietary fiber, which aids in preventing constipation, promoting regular bowel movements, and supporting a healthy weight.

By incorporating essential nutrients through raw foods into your diet can provide numerous health benefits. Whether you follow a raw vegan, raw paleo, raw fruitarian, raw juice, raw vegetarian, raw dairy-free, raw gluten-free, raw nut-based, raw alkaline, or raw superfood diet, the nutrient density of raw foods is unparalleled. By consuming raw foods, you can ensure that your body receives a wide array of vitamins, minerals, antioxidants, enzymes, and fiber, all of which are vital for supporting optimal health and well-being. So, embark on your raw food revolution today and experience the transformative power of nature's most nourishing gifts.

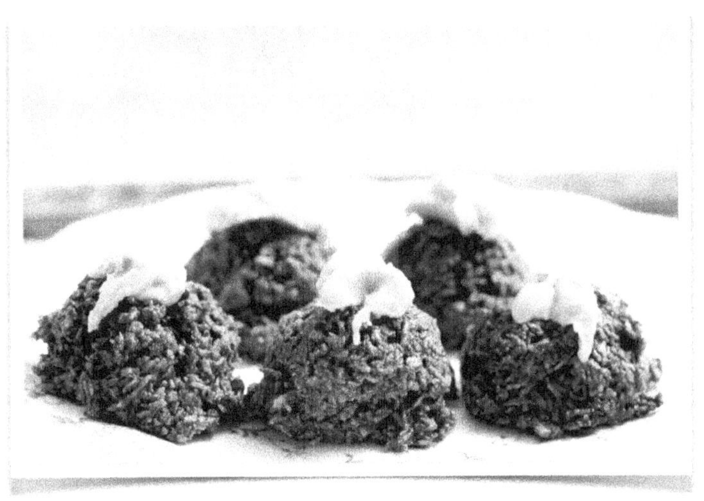

Raw Vegan Chocolate Macaroons

Chapter 5: The Raw Vegan Diet

The Raw Vegan Lifestyle is a powerful and transformative way of living that has gained significant popularity among health-conscious individuals. In this subchapter, we will delve into the depths of this lifestyle, unraveling its principles, benefits, and practical tips for incorporating it into your daily routine.

The concept of a raw vegan diet revolves around consuming uncooked and unprocessed plant-based foods. It excludes all animal products, including meat, dairy, eggs, and even honey. By embracing this lifestyle, you are not only nourishing your body with vibrant and nutrient-dense foods but also making a compassionate choice towards animals and the environment.

One of the key benefits of adopting a raw vegan diet is the abundance of enzymes, vitamins, and minerals present in raw plant foods. Cooking often depletes these vital nutrients, but by consuming them in their natural state, you are maximizing their nutritional value. This leads to increased energy levels, enhanced digestion, improved immunity, and overall vitality.

The raw vegan lifestyle encompasses various niches, each with its unique approach and focus. Whether you are interested in raw fruitarian, raw paleo, raw juice, raw vegetarian, or any other variation, this subchapter will provide you with a comprehensive understanding of each niche's principles and benefits. You will learn how to create a balanced and diverse raw vegan diet that suits your specific needs and preferences.

Incorporating the raw vegan lifestyle into your daily routine can initially seem overwhelming, but with proper guidance, it becomes an exciting and rewarding journey. This subchapter will provide you with practical tips on sourcing and selecting high-quality organic produce, preparing delicious and satisfying meals, and managing potential challenges such as social situations and traveling.

Furthermore, we will explore the wide range of health benefits associated with a raw vegan lifestyle. From weight loss and improved digestion to reduced risk of chronic diseases and enhanced mental clarity, this lifestyle can truly revolutionize your health and wellbeing.

Whether you are a seasoned raw food enthusiast or simply curious about the raw vegan lifestyle, this subchapter is your comprehensive guide to exploring and embracing this transformative way of living. Prepare to embark on a journey that will not only nourish your body but also inspire and empower you to make conscious choices for yourself, the animals, and the planet.

Nutritional Considerations for Raw Vegans

For health-conscious individuals following a raw vegan diet, understanding the nutritional considerations is essential to ensure a balanced and nourishing lifestyle. Raw veganism is a dietary choice that emphasizes the consumption of uncooked and unprocessed plant-based foods, avoiding all animal products. This subchapter will delve into the key nutritional considerations for raw vegans, exploring the various aspects of a well-rounded raw vegan diet.

One of the primary concerns for raw vegans is obtaining sufficient protein intake. While it is commonly believed that plant-based diets lack protein, this is a misconception. Raw vegans can obtain ample protein from sources such as leafy greens, nuts, seeds, and sprouted legumes.

Incorporating a variety of these protein-rich foods into meals and snacks is crucial for meeting daily protein requirements.

Another essential consideration is obtaining adequate amounts of essential fatty acids, particularly omega-3s. Raw vegans can obtain these healthy fats from sources like flaxseeds, chia seeds, hemp seeds, and walnuts. Including these foods regularly in the diet can help maintain optimal brain function, support heart health, and reduce inflammation.

Raw vegans should also pay attention to their vitamin and mineral intake. While plant-based foods are abundant in vitamins and minerals, certain nutrients may require special attention. For instance, vitamin B12, which is primarily found in animal products, can be challenging to obtain on a raw vegan diet. Supplementation or consumption of fortified foods may be necessary to ensure adequate levels of this essential vitamin.

Iron, calcium, and zinc are other nutrients that may require careful consideration for raw vegans. Leafy greens, seaweeds, nuts, and seeds are excellent sources of these minerals. However, it is essential to ensure proper absorption by pairing them with vitamin C-rich foods, like citrus fruits or bell peppers, which enhance mineral absorption.

Additionally, raw vegans should focus on consuming a wide variety of fruits and vegetables to ensure a well-rounded nutrient intake. Incorporating a rainbow of colors into meals ensures a diverse array of vitamins, minerals, antioxidants, and phytochemicals, promoting optimal health and wellbeing.

By adopting a raw vegan diet can be a highly nutritious and health-promoting choice. However, to ensure a well-balanced diet, raw vegans must pay attention to their protein, essential fatty acid, vitamin, and mineral intake. By incorporating a diverse range of plant-based foods and incorporating necessary supplements, raw vegans can thrive and enjoy the numerous benefits of this lifestyle.

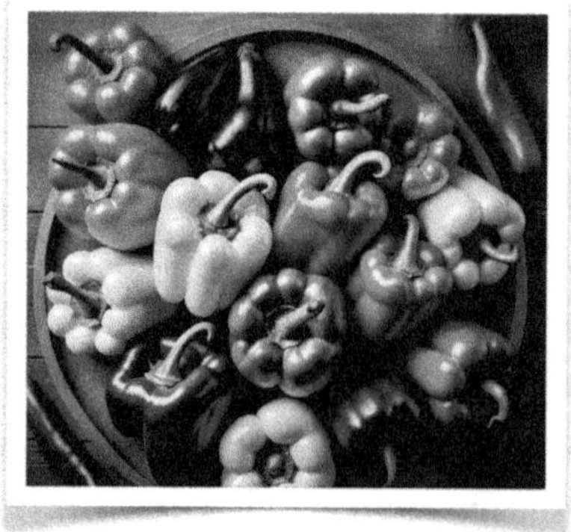

Chapter 6: The Raw Paleo Diet

Understanding the Raw Paleo Lifestyle

The raw paleo lifestyle is a unique approach to nutrition and well-being that combines the principles of the raw food diet with the principles of the paleo diet. It is a way of eating that focuses on consuming unprocessed, whole, and nutrient-dense foods in their natural state. This subchapter aims to provide a comprehensive understanding of the raw paleo lifestyle, its benefits, and how it can be incorporated into your daily routine.

The raw paleo lifestyle is based on the belief that our bodies are designed to thrive on the foods that our ancestors ate during the Paleolithic era. This means consuming foods that are free from additives, preservatives, and chemicals, and instead focusing on fresh fruits, vegetables, nuts, seeds, and lean meats. By consuming these foods in their raw, uncooked state, proponents of the raw paleo lifestyle believe that they are able to obtain the maximum amount of nutrients and enzymes from their food, leading to increased energy levels, improved digestion, and enhanced overall health.

One of the key principles of the raw paleo lifestyle is the concept of bioavailability. This refers to the body's ability to absorb and utilize the nutrients present in the food we eat. By consuming raw foods, we are able to preserve the natural enzymes and vitamins that are often destroyed during the cooking process. This means that our bodies can more effectively absorb and utilize the nutrients in our food, leading to improved digestion and nutrient absorption.

Another important aspect of the raw paleo lifestyle is the emphasis on consuming organic, locally sourced, and seasonal foods. This not only ensures that we are getting the highest quality produce but also supports local farmers and reduces our carbon footprint.

Incorporating the raw paleo lifestyle into your daily routine may require some adjustments, as it involves eliminating processed foods, grains, and dairy products. However, the benefits of this lifestyle are numerous. Many adherents report increased energy levels, improved digestion, weight loss, and a decreased risk of chronic diseases such as heart disease and diabetes.

The raw paleo lifestyle offers health-conscious individuals a unique and holistic approach to nutrition. By focusing on consuming raw, unprocessed, and nutrient-dense foods, we can optimize our health and well-being. Whether you choose to follow a raw vegan, raw fruitarian, raw juice, raw vegetarian, or any other variation of the raw paleo lifestyle, the key is to listen to your body and make choices that support your individual health goals.

Incorporating Raw Animal Products in Your Diet

For health-conscious individuals following a raw food diet, there are various approaches to consider, including the incorporation of raw animal products. While many people associate raw foodism with veganism or vegetarianism, it is important to remember that raw food diets can be tailored to individual preferences and nutritional needs. This subchapter aims to shed light on incorporating raw animal products into your diet while maintaining the principles of a health-conscious lifestyle.

The raw food revolution encompasses various niches, including the raw vegan diet, raw paleo diet, raw fruitarian diet, raw juice diet, raw vegetarian diet, raw dairy-free diet, raw gluten-free diet, raw nut-based diet, raw alkaline diet, and raw superfood diet. Each of these niches has its own unique approach, and the inclusion of raw animal products can be adapted accordingly.

When incorporating raw animal products into your diet, it is crucial to prioritize quality and sourcing. Opt for organic, wild-caught, and grass-fed options whenever possible. This ensures that you are consuming the highest quality animal products, free from harmful antibiotics, hormones, and other additives.

For those following a raw vegan or vegetarian diet, raw animal products may seem contradictory. However, it is important to remember that a health-conscious lifestyle is not about following strict rules but rather prioritizing optimal nutrition and overall well-being. If you choose to include raw animal products, options such as raw dairy, raw eggs, or raw fish can provide essential nutrients like protein, omega-3 fatty acids, and vitamin B12 that are often lacking in a plant-based diet.

For individuals following a raw paleo or raw fruitarian diet, incorporating raw animal products may be more aligned with their dietary principles.

Raw meat, such as carpaccio or tartare, can be consumed in moderation, taking into account the importance of sourcing high-quality, grass-fed, and organic options.

It is important to note that before making any significant changes to your diet, it is advisable to consult with a healthcare professional or registered dietitian. They can provide personalized guidance based on your nutritional needs and health goals.

In conclusion, incorporating raw animal products into your diet can be a valid choice for health-conscious individuals following various niches within the raw food revolution. By prioritizing quality sourcing and considering individual nutritional needs, raw animal products can provide an additional source of essential nutrients and enhance the diversity of your raw food repertoire. Remember, it is essential to listen to your body and make informed decisions that align with your personal health goals.

Raw Paleo Recipe Ideas

Let's explore a variety of delicious and nutritious raw paleo recipe ideas to help you embrace a healthy and natural lifestyle. Whether you follow a raw food, raw vegan, raw fruitarian, raw juice, raw vegetarian, raw dairy-free, raw gluten-free, raw nut-based, raw alkaline, or raw superfood diet, these recipes will provide you with plenty of options to satisfy your taste buds and nourish your body.

1. Raw Zucchini Noodles with Avocado Pesto: Replace traditional pasta with spiralized zucchini noodles and top them with a creamy avocado pesto sauce. This dish is packed with healthy fats and fiber, making it a perfect choice for those following a raw paleo or raw vegan diet.

2. Raw Cauliflower Rice Stir-Fry: Using a food processor, pulse cauliflower florets until they resemble rice grains. Sauté the cauliflower rice with your favorite vegetables, herbs, and spices. This dish is low in carbohydrates and ideal for those on a raw paleo or raw alkaline diet.

3. Raw Paleo Energy Balls: Combine dates, nuts, seeds, and cacao powder in a food processor. Roll the mixture into bite-sized energy balls and

refrigerate. These nutritious snacks are suitable for all raw diets, providing a quick boost of energy and essential nutrients.

4. Raw Fruit Parfait: Layer fresh seasonal fruits with coconut yogurt and raw nuts in a glass. This colorful and refreshing dessert is perfect for those following a raw fruitarian or raw dairy-free diet.

5. Raw Superfood Smoothie: Blend together your favorite leafy greens, berries, superfood powders, and a plant-based milk of your choice. This nutrient-dense smoothie is suitable for all raw diets, providing a quick and convenient way to nourish your body.

Remember, when following a raw paleo diet, it is essential to focus on consuming organic, unprocessed, and whole foods. Experiment with different combinations of fruits, vegetables, nuts, seeds, and herbs to create your own unique raw paleo recipes.

By incorporating these raw paleo recipe ideas into your daily routine, you can enjoy a wide variety of flavors while nourishing your body with the vital nutrients it needs. Embrace the raw food revolution and discover the incredible health benefits that come with it.

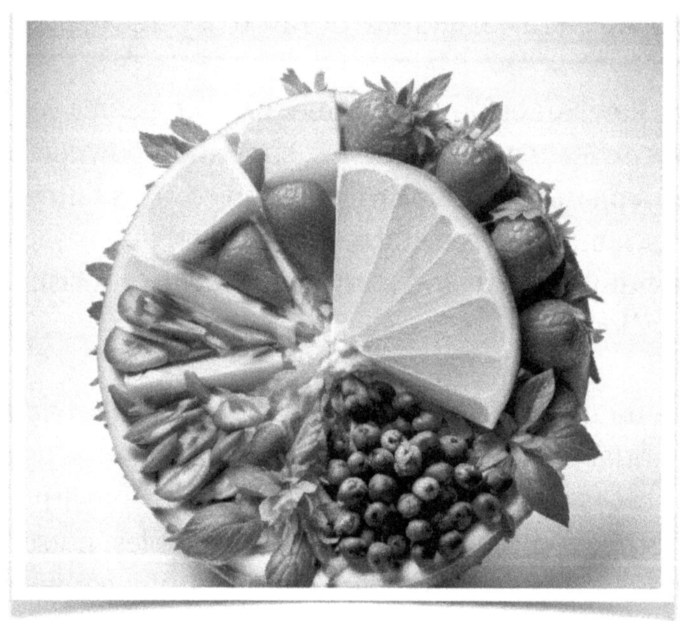

Chapter 7: The Raw Fruitarian Diet

Embracing the Fruitarian Lifestyle

In the world of health and wellness, there is a vast array of dietary choices available to individuals seeking optimal well-being. One such lifestyle that has gained significant attention and admiration is the fruitarian diet. Embracing the fruitarian lifestyle means adopting a diet primarily composed of fresh fruits, while also incorporating other raw plant-based foods.

The fruitarian diet is not just a trend; it is a philosophy that promotes harmony with nature and a deep connection with the earth. By consuming a diet rich in fruits, individuals can experience a myriad of health benefits, including increased energy levels, improved digestion, and enhanced mental clarity.

Fruits are nature's perfect food, packed with essential vitamins, minerals, and antioxidants. They provide the body with a plentiful supply of nutrients while simultaneously cleansing and detoxifying it.

The high water content in fruits aids in hydration, while their natural sugars provide a sustainable energy source.

By following a fruitarian diet, one can experience weight loss, improved skin complexion, and a strengthened immune system. Fruits are naturally low in calories and high in fiber, making them an ideal choice for those looking to shed excess pounds. Additionally, the abundance of antioxidants present in fruits helps combat free radicals and reduce the risk of chronic diseases.

The fruitarian lifestyle extends beyond just the physical aspect; it encompasses a spiritual connection with the earth and a deep appreciation for the natural world. By consuming foods in their raw, unprocessed form, individuals can tap into the life force energy present in nature. This energy not only nourishes the body but also uplifts the spirit, promoting a sense of vitality and well-being.

It is important to note that while the fruitarian lifestyle offers numerous benefits, it may not be suitable for everyone. Individuals with specific dietary needs or health conditions should consult with a healthcare professional before adopting this lifestyle.

Embracing the fruitarian lifestyle can be a transformative journey for health-conscious individuals seeking a natural and sustainable way of nourishing their bodies. By incorporating an abundance of fresh fruits and raw plant-based foods into their diet, individuals can experience enhanced vitality, improved well-being, and a deeper connection with the earth. So, why not take a bite into the sweet and vibrant world of the fruitarian lifestyle and embark on a path towards optimal health and wellness?

Meeting Nutritional Needs as a Fruitarian

As health-conscious individuals, we are constantly seeking ways to improve our well-being and nourish our bodies with the best possible fuel. One dietary approach gaining popularity among various niches, including raw food diet enthusiasts, raw vegan enthusiasts, and raw fruitarian devotees, is the raw fruitarian diet. In this subchapter, we will explore how to meet our nutritional needs while following a fruitarian lifestyle.

The raw fruitarian diet revolves around consuming predominantly fresh, raw fruits. While this diet may seem limited to some, it can provide an abundance of essential nutrients when properly planned and executed. Ensuring a balanced intake of macronutrients, vitamins, and minerals is crucial for optimal health.

First and foremost, it is important to include a variety of fruits in your daily diet. Different fruits offer distinct nutritional profiles, so incorporating a wide range ensures you receive a broad spectrum of vitamins and minerals. Citrus fruits, for instance, are rich in vitamin C, while bananas provide potassium and magnesium. Additionally, berries are packed with antioxidants, and tropical fruits like mangoes and papayas offer an array of vitamins.

To meet your protein requirements, incorporate protein-rich fruits such as avocados, durian, and coconuts into your meals. These fruits not only provide essential amino acids but also offer healthy fats, which are crucial for hormone production and overall well-being. Nuts and seeds can also be included for additional protein and healthy fats, while still adhering to the principles of a fruitarian diet.

Ensuring adequate intake of essential fatty acids is another important aspect of a fruitarian diet. While fruits are naturally low in fat, incorporating small amounts of avocados, coconuts, or nuts can provide the necessary omega-3 and omega-6 fatty acids. These fats support brain function, hormone production, and cardiovascular health.

Vitamin B12, which is primarily found in animal products, can be a concern for fruitarians. It is recommended to regularly monitor your B12 levels and consider supplementation if necessary. Additionally, incorporating seaweed, nutritional yeast, or fermented foods into your diet can provide some B12, although not in significant amounts.

To optimize mineral intake, it is essential to include a sufficient amount of leafy greens in your daily meals. Greens such as spinach, kale, and Swiss chard are rich in iron, calcium, and other minerals. Combining these greens with fruits in a variety of smoothies, salads, or juices can help meet your nutritional needs.

In conclusion, following a raw fruitarian diet can provide a plethora of health benefits when approached mindfully. By incorporating a wide variety of fruits, protein-rich foods, essential fatty acids, and mindful supplementation, you can ensure your nutritional needs are met while enjoying the

vibrant flavors and abundant health benefits of a
fruit-based lifestyle.

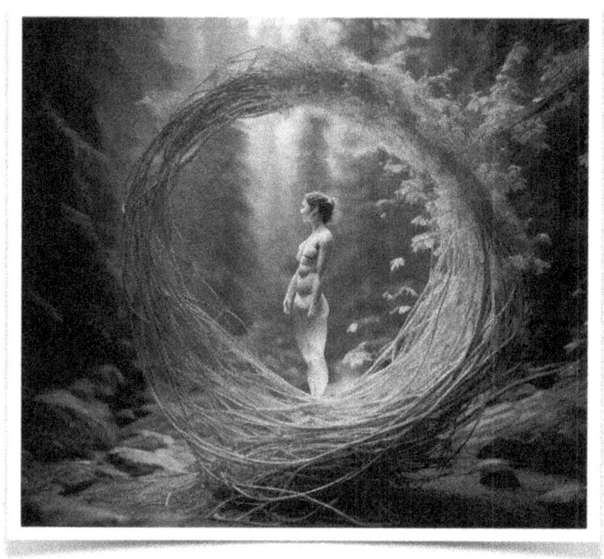

Chapter 8: The Raw Juice Diet

The Benefits of Juicing in a Raw Food Diet

Juicing has become increasingly popular among health-conscious individuals who follow a raw food diet. By extracting the nutrient-rich juice from fruits and vegetables, juicing offers a convenient and effective way to incorporate a wide variety of vitamins, minerals, and antioxidants into your daily routine. In this subchapter, we will explore the numerous benefits of juicing in a raw food diet and how it can contribute to overall health and well-being.

One of the primary advantages of juicing is the concentrated dose of nutrients it provides. When fruits and vegetables are juiced, their fibers are broken down, allowing the body to absorb the vitamins and minerals more efficiently. This means that even a small glass of juice can provide a significant amount of essential nutrients, helping to support a healthy immune system, improve digestion, and promote optimal organ function.

Additionally, juicing allows for easy consumption of a diverse range of fruits and vegetables. Many individuals struggle to consume the recommended daily servings of fruits and vegetables, but juicing offers a practical solution. By combining different ingredients, you can create delicious and nutritious juice blends that incorporate a wide array of vitamins, minerals, and antioxidants, all in one glass.

Another benefit of juicing is its potential to support detoxification. Raw fruits and vegetables are rich in enzymes that aid in the body's natural detoxification processes. By juicing, you can provide your body with a concentrated source of these enzymes, assisting in the removal of toxins and waste from the body.

Juicing can be an excellent way to increase hydration. Many fruits and vegetables have high water content, and juicing allows you to benefit from their hydrating properties. Proper hydration is essential for maintaining healthy skin, supporting digestion, and regulating body temperature.

For individuals following specific raw food diets, such as raw vegan, raw paleo, or raw fruitarian diets, juicing can be a valuable tool for meeting nutritional requirements. Juicing provides an efficient way to consume a wide variety of plant-based foods, ensuring a well-rounded intake of essential vitamins, minerals, and antioxidants.

Juicing offers a convenient and efficient way to consume a concentrated dose of nutrients, supports detoxification, increases hydration, and helps meet nutritional requirements for various raw food diets. By embracing juicing as part of your raw food journey, you can enhance your overall health and well-being.

Different Types of Raw Juice Diets

In the world of raw food diets, there are numerous options to explore, each offering unique benefits and approaches to health and wellness. Raw juice diets, in particular, have gained immense popularity among health-conscious individuals seeking to cleanse their bodies, boost energy levels, and improve overall vitality. In this subchapter, we will delve into the different types of raw juice diets, shedding light on the specific characteristics and advantages of each.

1. Raw Vegan Juice Diet: This diet focuses on consuming only plant-based juices, avoiding any

animal products. It is rich in vitamins, minerals, and antioxidants, promoting weight loss, increased energy, and improved digestion.

2. Raw Paleo Juice Diet: Combining the principles of the raw food diet with those of the paleo diet, this approach emphasizes consuming juices made from raw fruits, vegetables, and grass-fed or wild-caught meats. Advocates claim it helps maintain a lean physique, enhances mental clarity, and supports overall well-being.

3. Raw Fruitarian Juice Diet: This diet consists of consuming juices made exclusively from raw fruits, including berries, citrus fruits, and tropical varieties. It provides a burst of natural sugars, vitamins, and enzymes, aiding in detoxification, weight loss, and increased vitality.

4. Raw Vegetarian Juice Diet: Similar to the raw vegan juice diet, this approach allows for the inclusion of dairy products such as raw milk, cheese, and yogurt. It provides a wider range of nutrients while still promoting detoxification and overall health.

5. Raw Dairy-Free Juice Diet: Focusing on juices made solely from fruits and vegetables, this diet

excludes any dairy products. It is particularly beneficial for those with lactose intolerance or dairy allergies, supporting digestion, reducing inflammation, and enhancing vitality.

6. Raw Gluten-Free Juice Diet: This diet eliminates gluten-containing ingredients such as wheat, barley, and rye, while incorporating a variety of raw juices. It is ideal for individuals with gluten sensitivities or celiac disease, promoting gut health, weight loss, and increased energy levels.

7. Raw Nut-Based Juice Diet: This diet incorporates juices made from a combination of raw fruits and vegetables alongside various nuts and seeds. It provides essential fatty acids, proteins, and fiber, supporting brain function, muscle recovery, and overall well-being.

8. Raw Alkaline Juice Diet: This diet focuses on consuming juices that alkalize the body, balancing pH levels and reducing acidity. It enhances detoxification, boosts energy, and supports optimal organ function.

9. Raw Superfood Juice Diet: This diet combines raw juices with nutrient-dense superfoods like spirulina, chlorella, wheatgrass, and maca. It

maximizes nutrient absorption, strengthens the immune system, and promotes overall vitality.

Chapter 9: The Raw Vegetarian Diet

Exploring the Raw Vegetarian Lifestyle

In recent years, there has been a significant increase in the number of health-conscious individuals embracing the raw vegetarian lifestyle. This subchapter aims to provide a comprehensive guide for those who wish to embark on this transformative journey towards optimal health and wellness.

The raw vegetarian diet is a plant-based eating plan that emphasizes the consumption of unprocessed, uncooked fruits, vegetables, nuts, seeds, and sprouted grains. By excluding all animal products, including dairy, this diet offers a plethora of health benefits and is popular among individuals seeking weight loss, increased energy levels, and improved digestion.

One of the key advantages of the raw vegetarian diet is its abundance of vitamins, minerals, and antioxidants. Raw fruits and vegetables are packed with essential nutrients that are often lost during the cooking process. By consuming these foods in their natural state, health-conscious individuals can ensure they are getting the most out of their meals, supporting their immune system, and promoting overall well-being.

Another intriguing aspect of the raw vegetarian lifestyle is the focus on alkaline-forming foods. By consuming a predominantly alkaline diet, individuals can reduce the acidity in their bodies and promote a more balanced pH level. This is believed to help prevent and combat diseases, boost energy levels, and improve overall vitality.

For those concerned about meeting their protein needs on a raw vegetarian diet, fear not. There are plenty of plant-based sources of protein available, including nuts, seeds, legumes, and sprouted grains. These protein-rich foods can provide the necessary amino acids for muscle repair, growth, and overall body function.

To successfully adopt and thrive on a raw vegetarian diet, it is important to experiment with different recipes and meal plans. This subchapter provides a range of delicious and creative ideas to help you incorporate raw vegetarian meals into your daily routine. From refreshing salads and zoodles to delectable smoothie bowls and raw desserts, there is a wealth of culinary possibilities waiting to be explored.

In conclusion, the raw vegetarian lifestyle offers health-conscious individuals an opportunity to explore a plant-based, uncooked diet that can enhance overall well-being. By focusing on nutrient-dense, alkaline-forming foods, individuals can experience increased energy levels, improved digestion, and enhanced vitality. So, whether you are interested in the raw fruitarian diet, raw vegan diet, or any other variation, this subchapter will serve as a comprehensive guide to help you embark on your raw food revolution.

Balancing Nutrients as a Raw Vegetarian

As health-conscious individuals, we understand the importance of nourishing our bodies with wholesome foods. One dietary approach that has gained significant popularity among health enthusiasts is the raw vegetarian diet. This subchapter will explore the principles of balancing nutrients while following a raw vegetarian lifestyle, catering to the various niches of the raw food revolution.

The raw vegetarian diet emphasizes the consumption of unprocessed, plant-based foods in their natural state. This includes fruits, vegetables, nuts, seeds, and sprouted grains. While this diet offers numerous health benefits, ensuring proper nutrient balance is crucial for optimal well-being.

One key aspect of maintaining nutrient balance as a raw vegetarian is to consume a wide variety of fruits and vegetables. Different fruits and vegetables offer unique nutritional profiles, so including a rainbow of colors on your plate ensures a diverse range of vitamins, minerals, and phytonutrients. Incorporating leafy greens such as kale, spinach, and Swiss chard provides essential nutrients like iron, calcium, and vitamin K.

Protein is an essential macronutrient, and as a raw vegetarian, it's important to ensure an adequate intake. While fruits and vegetables contain some protein, incorporating plant-based protein sources like nuts, seeds, and legumes is essential. Sprouted legumes, such as lentils and chickpeas, are particularly beneficial as they enhance the bioavailability of nutrients and are easier to digest.

Raw vegetarians should also pay attention to their omega-3 fatty acid intake. While many people rely on fish as their primary source of omega-3s, raw vegetarians can obtain these essential fats from sources like chia seeds, flaxseeds, and walnuts. These foods are not only rich in omega-3s but also provide fiber and other important nutrients.

Another key consideration for raw vegetarians is vitamin B12. Since this vitamin is primarily found in animal products, it's crucial to ensure adequate intake through fortified foods or supplements. Nutritional yeast is a popular option as it provides a cheesy flavor and is often fortified with vitamin B12.

Lastly, raw vegetarians should be mindful of their calcium intake. While dairy is not consumed on this diet, there are plenty of plant-based sources of calcium available. Sesame seeds, leafy greens, almonds, and fortified plant-based milk alternatives are excellent choices to meet your calcium needs.

In conclusion, following a raw vegetarian diet can provide numerous health benefits. By incorporating a diverse range of fruits, vegetables, nuts, seeds, and legumes, you can ensure a balanced intake of essential nutrients. Paying attention to protein sources, omega-3 fatty acids, vitamin B12, and calcium will help you thrive on this health-conscious dietary path.

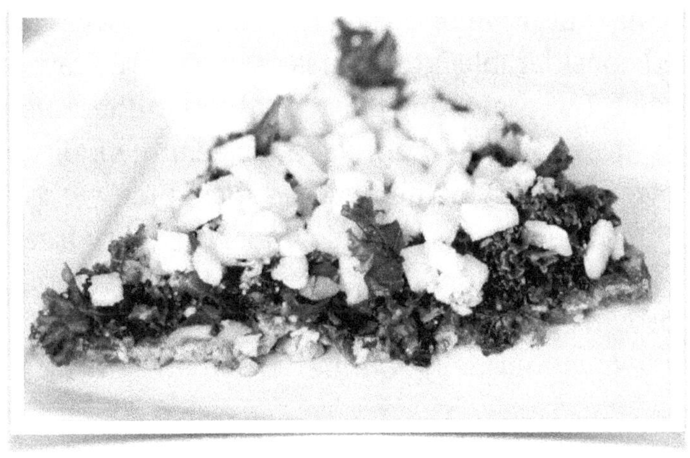

Raw Maui Waui Pizza
Gorilla Food in Vancouver

Chapter 10: The Raw Dairy-Free Diet

Understanding Dairy-Free Raw Food Choices
In recent years, the popularity of raw food diets has soared among health-conscious individuals seeking to optimize their well-being and vitality. One particular variation of this dietary approach that has gained considerable attention is the dairy-free raw food diet. By eliminating dairy products, adherents to this lifestyle aim to improve their health, vitality, and overall quality of life. In this subchapter, we will delve into the reasons behind choosing a dairy-free raw food diet, explore the various benefits it offers, and provide practical tips for incorporating this lifestyle into your daily routine.

The decision to embrace a dairy-free raw food diet stems from a multitude of reasons. Firstly, many individuals struggle with lactose intolerance or dairy allergies, making it necessary to avoid dairy products altogether. Secondly, dairy consumption has been linked to various health concerns, including inflammation, digestive issues, and compromised immune function. By eliminating dairy, individuals can alleviate these symptoms and experience enhanced well-being. Additionally, the ethical and environmental concerns surrounding conventional dairy production have prompted many health-conscious individuals to seek alternative options.

So, what are the benefits of embarking on a dairy-free raw food diet? Firstly, this dietary approach is abundant in fresh fruits, vegetables, nuts, seeds, and sprouted grains, providing a rich source of essential nutrients, antioxidants, and enzymes. By consuming these raw, unprocessed foods, individuals can optimize their nutrient intake and support overall health. Moreover, a dairy-free raw food diet can often lead to weight loss, increased energy levels, improved digestion, and enhanced mental clarity. The elimination of dairy products can also alleviate skin issues, such as acne and eczema, and reduce the risk of chronic diseases, including heart disease and diabetes.

Incorporating a dairy-free raw food diet into your daily routine may seem daunting at first, but with a few practical tips, it can become an enjoyable and sustainable lifestyle choice. Start by gradually reducing your dairy intake and replacing it with plant-based alternatives such as almond milk, coconut yogurt, or cashew cheese. Experiment with new recipes and explore the wide range of fruits, vegetables, nuts, and seeds available to create delicious and satisfying meals. It is also essential to ensure you are meeting your nutritional needs by incorporating a variety of foods and considering supplements such as vitamin B12 and omega-3 fatty acids.

Understanding the principles and benefits of a dairy-free raw food diet is crucial for health-conscious individuals seeking optimal well-being. By embracing this lifestyle, individuals can experience improved health, increased energy, and a reduced risk of chronic disease. With careful planning and a willingness to explore new culinary horizons, adopting a dairy-free raw food diet can be a transformative and rewarding journey towards vibrant health and vitality.

Navigating Dairy Alternatives in a Raw Food Diet
Introduction:

For health-conscious individuals following a raw food diet, finding suitable dairy alternatives can be a challenge. Many traditional dairy products are excluded from this way of eating, but fear not! This subchapter will guide you through the world of dairy alternatives, providing options that align with various raw food diets such as raw vegan, raw paleo, raw fruitarian, raw juice, raw vegetarian, raw dairy-free, raw gluten-free, raw nut-based, raw alkaline, and raw superfood diets.

Exploring Dairy-Free Alternatives:

One of the key aspects of raw food diets is the exclusion of dairy products, which can be a source of inflammation and discomfort for many individuals. However, there are numerous dairy alternatives available that can be incorporated into your raw food journey. These alternatives not only provide essential nutrients but also offer satisfying flavors and textures.

Plant-Based "Milks":

Plant-based milks like almond, coconut, and cashew milk have become increasingly popular among raw food enthusiasts. These dairy alternatives are rich in vitamins, minerals, and healthy fats. They can be used as a base for smoothies, poured over raw granolas, or added to raw dessert recipes to provide a creamy texture.

Raw Cheese Substitutes:

If you're missing the creamy goodness of cheese, fear not! Raw food diets offer a plethora of dairy-free cheese alternatives made from nuts, seeds, and even vegetables. These delicious substitutes can be used in various recipes, including raw lasagna, pizzas, and salads, providing a similar taste and texture to traditional cheese.

Yogurt Alternatives:

For those who enjoy the tangy delight of yogurt, raw food diets offer a range of options. Fermented nut and seed-based yogurts provide probiotics and enzymes, promoting a healthy gut. These yogurts can be enjoyed plain or mixed with raw fruits and superfoods for a nutrient-dense breakfast or snack.

Butter and Cream Replacements:

Raw food diets also provide alternatives to butter and cream. Coconut oil and avocado are excellent choices for spreading on raw bread or adding to recipes that require a creamy texture. Additionally, nut-based creams made from cashews or macadamia nuts can be used in savory or sweet dishes, adding richness and flavor.

Navigating dairy alternatives in a raw food diet doesn't mean sacrificing taste or nutrition. By exploring the wide range of dairy-free options available, you can create delicious and satisfying meals that align with your chosen raw food diet. Whether you follow a raw vegan, raw paleo, raw fruitarian, or any other raw food niche, incorporating these dairy alternatives will enhance your culinary experience while keeping you healthy and vibrant.

Chapter 11: The Raw Gluten-Free Diet

Embracing a Gluten-Free Lifestyle in Raw Food

Living a gluten-free lifestyle has become increasingly popular in recent years, with more and more individuals recognizing the detrimental effects that gluten can have on their health. For those following a raw food diet, adopting a gluten-free approach can be an excellent way to further enhance overall well-being and reap the numerous benefits that come with a gluten-free lifestyle.

The raw food movement, which encompasses various niches such as the raw vegan, raw paleo, raw fruitarian, raw juice, raw vegetarian, raw dairy-free, raw nut-based, raw alkaline, and raw superfood diets, promotes the consumption of unprocessed and uncooked foods in their most natural state. By eliminating gluten from this equation, individuals can experience heightened energy levels, improved digestion, and enhanced overall vitality.

Gluten, a protein found in wheat, barley, and rye, can often lead to inflammation in the body, causing discomfort and digestive issues for many individuals. By adhering to a gluten-free raw food diet, individuals can avoid this potential source of inflammation, allowing their bodies to function optimally.

In the realm of raw food, there is an abundance of gluten-free options available. Nut-based flours, such as almond or coconut flour, can be used as substitutes for traditional gluten-containing flours in recipes. Gluten-free grains, such as quinoa or buckwheat, can be sprouted and incorporated into a variety of dishes. Additionally, fruits and vegetables provide an array of gluten-free options, allowing for endless creativity in meal preparation.

By embracing a gluten-free lifestyle within the realm of raw food, individuals can experience a myriad of health benefits. Increased energy levels, improved digestion, clearer skin, and weight loss are just a few of the advantages that can be enjoyed. Additionally, a gluten-free raw food diet can be an effective approach for those with gluten sensitivities or celiac disease, as it eliminates the need for gluten-containing foods altogether.

For health-conscious individuals following a raw food diet, embracing a gluten-free lifestyle can be a powerful way to optimize well-being. By eliminating gluten from their diet, individuals can experience improved digestion, increased energy, and enhanced overall vitality. With a wide range of gluten-free options available within the raw food movement, it has never been easier to embark on this exciting journey towards better health.

Finding Gluten-Free Alternatives in a Raw Diet

For health-conscious individuals following a raw food diet, it is important to identify and incorporate gluten-free alternatives into their meal plans. Gluten, a protein found in wheat, barley, and rye, can cause digestive issues and inflammation in some individuals. Fortunately, there are numerous gluten-free options available within the realm of raw food diets.

One of the primary considerations when seeking gluten-free alternatives in a raw diet is to focus on whole, unprocessed foods. Choosing fresh fruits, vegetables, nuts, and seeds eliminates the risk of gluten contamination. These natural foods are not only gluten-free but also provide essential vitamins, minerals, and antioxidants.

Raw fruits and vegetables can serve as the foundation of a gluten-free raw diet. Incorporating a variety of colorful produce ensures a wide range of nutrients while adding flavor and texture to your meals. From leafy greens like spinach and kale to vibrant berries and tropical fruits, the options are endless.

Nuts and seeds are another valuable component of a gluten-free raw diet. Almonds, cashews, walnuts, and chia seeds are excellent sources of healthy fats, protein, and fiber. They can be used to make nut-based milks, spreads, and even gluten-free crackers or breads.

In addition to whole foods, there are specific gluten-free substitutes that can be used in raw food dishes. For instance, coconut flour, almond flour, and flaxseed meal can be used as replacements for traditional wheat flour. These alternatives not only eliminate gluten but also add a distinctive flavor and texture to raw desserts or breads.

Another option is to explore gluten-free grains such as quinoa, buckwheat, and amaranth. While these grains are not typically consumed in their raw form, they can be sprouted or soaked to increase their nutritional value and digestibility.

When preparing raw meals, it is important to read labels and check for potential sources of hidden gluten. Some products may contain gluten-based additives, so it is essential to choose certified gluten-free options or make your own from scratch.

Following a gluten-free raw diet is achievable and beneficial for health-conscious individuals. By focusing on whole, unprocessed foods, incorporating a variety of fruits, vegetables, nuts, and seeds, and exploring alternative flours and grains, individuals can enjoy a diverse range of gluten-free options within their raw food diet. Remember to always read labels and choose certified gluten-free products to ensure a truly gluten-free experience.

Gluten-Free Raw Food Recipe Ideas

For health-conscious individuals following various raw food diets, it can sometimes be challenging to find delicious and creative gluten-free recipes. However, with a little inspiration and experimentation, you can enjoy a wide range of gluten-free raw food dishes that are both nutritious and satisfying. In this subchapter, we will explore some fantastic gluten-free raw food recipe ideas that cater to different raw food diets, ensuring everyone can find something that suits their preferences.

1. Raw Vegan Zucchini Noodles with Avocado Pesto:
Swap out traditional pasta for zucchini noodles and top them with a creamy avocado pesto sauce. This simple yet flavorful dish is packed with nutrients and healthy fats.

2. Raw Paleo Cauliflower Rice Stir-Fry:
Using cauliflower as a rice substitute, create a delicious stir-fry with your favorite vegetables and a tangy sauce. This recipe provides a grain-free option for those following a raw paleo diet.

3. Raw Fruitarian Breakfast Parfait:

Start your day with a refreshing and nutritious fruit parfait. Layer different types of fruits, raw nuts, and seeds, and top with a dairy-free yogurt alternative for a satisfying and energizing breakfast.

4. Raw Juice Diet Green Smoothie:
Blend together a variety of leafy greens, cucumber, celery, and your choice of fruits to create a vibrant and nutrient-packed green smoothie. This recipe is perfect for those following a raw juice diet.

5. Raw Vegetarian Nori Wraps:
Wrap fresh vegetables, sprouts, and avocado in nori seaweed sheets for a satisfying and light meal. This recipe is ideal for raw vegetarians looking for a quick and easy lunch option.

6. Raw Dairy-Free Chocolate Mousse:
Indulge in a rich and creamy chocolate mousse made with avocados, raw cacao powder, and a natural sweetener of your choice. This dessert is perfect for those following a raw dairy-free diet.

7. Raw Nut-Based Energy Bars:

Create your own gluten-free energy bars using a variety of raw nuts, dried fruits, and superfoods like chia seeds or hemp hearts. These bars make for a convenient and nutritious snack on the go.

8. Raw Alkaline Green Salad:
Combine a variety of alkaline vegetables such as kale, spinach, cucumber, and bell peppers to create a refreshing and detoxifying green salad. This recipe is suitable for those following a raw alkaline diet.

9. Raw Superfood Smoothie Bowl:
Blend together your favorite superfoods like spirulina, maca powder, and goji berries with frozen fruits and a liquid of your choice. Pour it into a bowl and top with fresh fruits, nuts, and seeds for a vibrant and nutrient-dense breakfast or snack.

10. Raw Gluten-Free Pizza with a Nut-Based Crust:
Make a gluten-free pizza crust using a combination of raw nuts, seeds, and herbs. Top it with your favorite raw vegetables, herbs, and a delicious tomato sauce for a satisfying gluten-free pizza experience.

With these gluten-free raw food recipe ideas, you can explore the world of raw food cuisine while catering to your specific dietary needs. Whether you follow a raw vegan, raw paleo, raw fruitarian, or any other raw food diet, these recipes will surely delight your taste buds and contribute to your overall health and well-being.

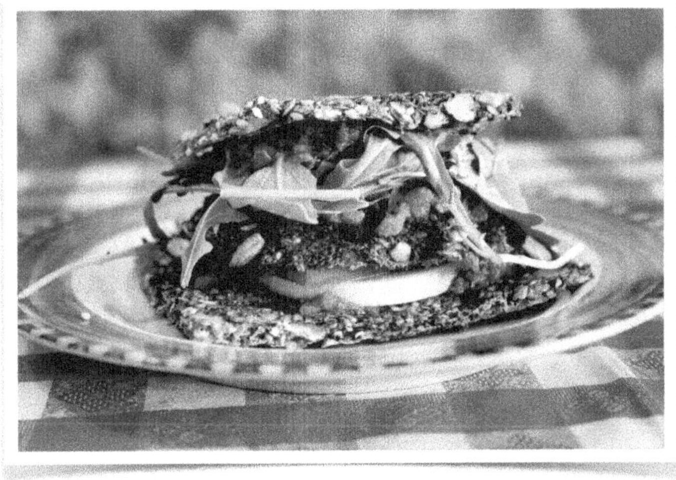

Raw Vegan Veggy Patty

Chapter 12: The Raw Nut-Based Diet

Incorporating Nut-Based Foods in a Raw Diet

Nuts are a powerhouse of nutrition and incorporating them into a raw diet can greatly enhance its health benefits. Whether you follow a raw vegan, raw paleo, raw fruitarian, raw juice, raw vegetarian, raw dairy-free, raw gluten-free, raw alkaline, raw superfood, or any other raw diet, nuts can be a valuable addition to your meal plan.

Nuts are packed with essential nutrients such as healthy fats, protein, fiber, vitamins, and minerals. They provide a sustainable source of energy and help maintain a feeling of fullness, making them an excellent choice for those looking to manage their weight. Furthermore, nuts contain antioxidants that protect the body against cell damage and reduce the risk of chronic diseases.

One of the simplest ways to incorporate nuts into a raw diet is by using them as a base for delicious nut butters. Almond butter, cashew butter, and walnut butter are just a few examples that can be easily made at home using a food processor or blender. These nut butters can be spread on raw crackers, vegetables, or fruits for a quick and satisfying snack.

Another great way to enjoy nuts in a raw diet is by making raw nut milk. Nut milk can be made by blending soaked nuts with water and straining the mixture to remove any solids. This creamy and nutritious milk can be used as a base for smoothies, poured over raw granola, or enjoyed on its own.

Nuts can also be used to add texture and flavor to raw desserts. From raw cheesecakes and energy balls to nut-based crusts for pies, the possibilities are endless. By combining nuts with dates or other dried fruits, you can create healthy and indulgent treats that will satisfy your sweet tooth without compromising your raw diet.

Incorporating nut-based foods into a raw diet is a fantastic way to boost nutrition and add variety to your meals. Whether you choose to enjoy them as nut butters, nut milk, or in raw desserts, nuts provide a wealth of health benefits that cater to the diverse needs of health-conscious individuals following various raw diets. So go ahead and explore the world of nuts, and unlock the full potential of your raw food revolution.

Nutritional Benefits of Raw Nuts and Seeds

Raw nuts and seeds are nutritional powerhouses that offer a wide range of health benefits. Whether you follow a raw food diet, raw vegan diet, raw paleo diet, raw fruitarian diet, raw juice diet, raw vegetarian diet, raw dairy-free diet, raw gluten-free diet, raw nut-based diet, raw alkaline diet, or raw superfood diet, incorporating raw nuts and seeds into your daily routine can greatly enhance your overall well-being.

First and foremost, raw nuts and seeds are excellent sources of healthy fats. They contain essential fatty acids such as omega-3 and omega-6, which are crucial for brain function, hormone production, and heart health. These fats also help to reduce inflammation in the body, promote healthy skin, and support a strong immune system.

Additionally, raw nuts and seeds are rich in protein, making them an excellent choice for those following a plant-based diet. They provide all the essential amino acids necessary for muscle growth and repair, making them a perfect post-workout snack. Moreover, the high protein content in nuts and seeds helps to keep you feeling full and satisfied, reducing the temptation to indulge in unhealthy snacks.

Raw nuts and seeds are also packed with vitamins and minerals. They are particularly high in vitamin E, which is a powerful antioxidant that protects cells from damage caused by free radicals. They also contain an array of B vitamins, magnesium, zinc, iron, and calcium, all of which are essential for optimal health.

Furthermore, raw nuts and seeds are a great source of dietary fiber. Fiber plays a crucial role in maintaining a healthy digestive system and preventing constipation. It also helps to regulate blood sugar levels, lower cholesterol, and support weight management.

Incorporating raw nuts and seeds into your diet is incredibly easy. They can be enjoyed as a standalone snack, added to smoothies, sprinkled on top of salads or oatmeal, or used as a base for homemade energy bars. With such versatility, it's effortless to incorporate these nutrient-dense foods into your daily meals.

In conclusion, raw nuts and seeds are a valuable addition to any health-conscious individual's diet.

They offer a wide range of nutritional benefits, including healthy fats, protein, vitamins, minerals, and fiber. By incorporating these nutrient-dense foods into your daily routine, you can enhance your overall well-being and support your specific dietary needs, whether you follow a raw food diet, raw vegan diet, raw paleo diet, raw fruitarian diet, raw juice diet, raw vegetarian diet, raw dairy-free diet, raw gluten-free diet, raw nut-based diet, raw alkaline diet, or raw superfood diet.

Delicious Nut-Based Raw Food Recipes

If you are someone who follows a raw food diet or any of its variations like raw vegan, raw paleo, raw fruitarian, raw juice, raw vegetarian, raw dairy-free, raw gluten-free, raw nut-based, raw alkaline, or raw superfood diet, you probably already know the incredible health benefits of eating raw, natural foods. And what better way to enjoy the goodness of raw food than by incorporating delicious nut-based recipes into your diet?

Nuts are not only packed with essential nutrients and healthy fats, but they also add a rich and satisfying flavor to any dish. Whether you're looking for a quick snack, a hearty main course, or a delectable dessert, these nut-based raw food recipes are sure to tantalize your taste buds and nourish your body.

1. Raw Almond Milk Smoothie: Start your day right with a creamy and refreshing smoothie made from homemade almond milk, ripe bananas, and a handful of your favorite berries. This nutrient-packed beverage will keep you energized and satisfied throughout the morning.

2. Raw Walnut Taco Meat: Craving a savory and satisfying meal? Try this raw walnut taco meat recipe, made from soaked walnuts, sun-dried tomatoes, and a blend of spices. Serve it in lettuce wraps or atop a bed of zucchini noodles for a truly raw and delicious twist on a classic favorite.

3. Raw Cashew Cheesecake: Indulge your sweet tooth with a guilt-free dessert that will leave you wanting more. This raw cashew cheesecake is made from soaked cashews, dates, and coconut oil, blended until smooth and creamy. Top it with fresh berries or a drizzle of raw honey for an extra touch of decadence.

4. Raw Pecan Energy Balls: Need a quick and nutritious snack on the go? These raw pecan energy balls are the perfect solution. Made from a mixture

of pecans, dates, coconut flakes, and a hint of cinnamon, they are packed with natural sweetness and a satisfying crunch.

5. Raw Hazelnut Chocolate Spread: Looking for a healthier alternative to store-bought chocolate spreads? This raw hazelnut chocolate spread is a game-changer. Made from a combination of hazelnuts, raw cacao powder, and a touch of maple syrup, it's a rich and creamy treat that can be enjoyed on fruit, crackers, or straight from the spoon.

These are just a few examples of the countless nut-based raw food recipes you can enjoy on your journey towards optimal health. Experiment with different nuts, flavors, and textures to find your own favorites. Remember, eating raw doesn't mean sacrificing taste or satisfaction - it's about nourishing your body with wholesome, unprocessed foods that leave you feeling vibrant and alive. So go ahead, embrace the raw food revolution and discover the delicious possibilities that await you!

Chapter 13: The Raw Alkaline Diet

Understanding the Alkaline-Acid Balance in Raw Food

In the world of raw food diets, there is a key concept that health-conscious individuals need to grasp - the alkaline-acid balance. Raw food enthusiasts advocate for a diet that is rich in alkaline-forming foods to maintain optimal health and vitality. This subchapter will delve into the importance of understanding the alkaline-acid balance in raw food and how it can benefit those following various raw food diets.

The alkaline-acid balance refers to the pH levels in our bodies. pH stands for potential hydrogen and measures the acidity or alkalinity of a substance. The pH scale ranges from 0 to 14, with 7 being neutral. A pH below 7 is considered acidic, while a pH above 7 is alkaline. Our bodies function best when the pH levels are slightly alkaline, around 7.4.

Raw food diets, such as raw vegan, raw paleo, raw fruitarian, and others, emphasize consuming foods that promote an alkaline environment in the body. This is because many health issues, such as inflammation, weakened immune system, and chronic diseases, are believed to thrive in an acidic environment. By eating a predominantly alkaline diet, individuals can help maintain the body's pH balance and promote overall health.

Alkaline-forming foods include fresh fruits, vegetables, sprouts, nuts, and seeds. These foods are rich in essential vitamins, minerals, and antioxidants that support the body's natural detoxification processes and boost overall immunity. They also help maintain healthy bones, improve digestion, and provide long-lasting energy.

On the other hand, acid-forming foods, such as processed foods, animal products, refined sugars, and caffeine, contribute to acidity in the body. These foods can lead to inflammation, digestive issues, and decreased energy levels.

Understanding the alkaline-acid balance is crucial for health-conscious individuals following specific raw food diets. For example, those on a raw gluten-free diet can incorporate alkaline-forming foods like quinoa, amaranth, and buckwheat into their meals to maintain the pH balance. Similarly, raw dairy-free diet enthusiasts can focus on alkaline foods like leafy greens, avocados, and raw nuts to support their dietary needs.

The alkaline-acid balance plays a vital role in maintaining optimal health for individuals following various raw food diets. By consuming a predominantly alkaline diet rich in fresh fruits, vegetables, nuts, and seeds, individuals can create an alkaline environment in their bodies, supporting overall well-being. Understanding this balance allows health-conscious people to make informed choices when selecting their raw food ingredients and designing their meal plans.

Incorporating Alkaline-Rich Foods in Your Diet

For health-conscious individuals following various raw food diets such as raw vegan, raw paleo, raw fruitarian, raw juice, raw vegetarian, raw dairy-free, raw gluten-free, raw nut-based, raw alkaline, or raw superfood diet, understanding the importance of incorporating alkaline-rich foods is key to maintaining optimal health and vitality.

The concept of an alkaline diet revolves around the pH scale, which measures the acidity or alkalinity of a substance. The human body functions best when it is slightly alkaline, around 7.4 on the pH scale. Unfortunately, many modern diets consist of highly acidic foods, such as processed foods, sugar, caffeine, and animal products, which can lead to imbalances in the body and various health issues.

To counteract the acidity, incorporating alkaline-rich foods into your diet is crucial. These foods can help restore balance, improve digestion, boost energy levels, enhance immune function, and support overall well-being. Including a variety of alkaline-rich foods ensures that your body receives the necessary nutrients for optimal health.

Leafy green vegetables are excellent sources of alkaline-rich nutrients. Incorporate vegetables like kale, spinach, Swiss chard, and collard greens into your daily meals. These greens are not only packed with essential vitamins, minerals, and antioxidants but are also highly alkalizing.

Another alkaline food group to include is fresh fruits. While some fruits like lemons and grapefruits may seem acidic, they have an alkalizing effect on the body once digested. Opt for fruits such as watermelon, bananas, avocados, and berries to boost your alkaline intake.

Nuts and seeds are also an important part of an alkaline diet. Almonds, hemp seeds, chia seeds, and flaxseeds are all excellent choices. These nutrient-dense foods provide healthy fats, protein, and fiber while maintaining an alkaline balance in the body.

In addition to these food groups, incorporating alkaline-forming beverages such as herbal teas, green juices, and alkaline water can further support your body's pH balance.

By incorporating alkaline-rich foods into your daily meals, you can enhance the benefits of your chosen raw food diet. Remember to maintain variety and balance in your diet to ensure you are receiving a wide range of nutrients.

Embracing an alkaline diet can have a transformative effect on your health, allowing you to thrive on your raw food journey. Start incorporating these alkaline-rich foods today and experience the power of optimal nutrition for a vibrant and healthy life.

Chapter 14: The Raw Superfood Diet

Exploring the Power of Superfoods in a Raw Diet

In recent years, the concept of a raw food diet has gained significant attention among health-conscious individuals seeking to optimize their well-being. This revolutionary approach to nutrition emphasizes the consumption of unprocessed, uncooked, and predominantly plant-based foods. Within this realm, a subcategory has emerged that takes the raw food diet to a whole new level - the incorporation of superfoods.

Superfoods are nutrient-dense foods that are exceptionally beneficial for our health. They are packed with vitamins, minerals, antioxidants, and phytonutrients that can support optimal bodily functions and help prevent disease. When combined with a raw food diet, the power of superfoods is further amplified, offering a plethora of health benefits.

One of the key advantages of incorporating superfoods into a raw diet is their ability to enhance the overall nutritional value of meals. By adding nutrient-dense superfoods like spirulina, chia seeds, and goji berries to your raw dishes, you are increasing the intake of essential vitamins and minerals that are often lacking in a conventional diet. This boost in nutrition can help improve energy levels, promote healthy digestion, and support a strong immune system.

Furthermore, superfoods are renowned for their potent antioxidant properties. Antioxidants help combat free radicals in the body, which are unstable molecules that can cause cellular damage and contribute to the development of chronic diseases. By consuming antioxidant-rich superfoods such as blueberries, kale, and cacao, individuals on a raw diet can effectively reduce oxidative stress and promote long-term health.

Superfoods also offer unique health benefits specific to various niches within the raw food community. For those following a raw vegan diet, superfoods like hemp seeds and nutritional yeast can provide essential amino acids and vitamin B12. Raw paleo enthusiasts can benefit from superfoods like grass-fed beef liver and wild-caught fish, which are rich in omega-3 fatty acids and essential nutrients. Raw fruitarians can explore superfoods like acai berries and pitaya, while raw juice enthusiasts can incorporate wheatgrass and turmeric into their blends.

Incorporating superfoods into a raw diet can revolutionize your health and well-being. By harnessing the power of nutrient-dense foods, individuals can optimize their nutrition, boost their antioxidant intake, and reap the unique benefits aligned with their chosen raw food niche. So, whether you follow a raw vegan, raw paleo, raw fruitarian, or any other raw food diet, consider exploring the diverse world of superfoods and unlock their potential to revolutionize your health.

In today's fast-paced world, where processed and unhealthy foods dominate the market, it has become increasingly important to prioritize our health and well-being. For health-conscious individuals, embracing a raw food lifestyle can provide numerous benefits, including increased energy, improved digestion, weight loss, and a strengthened immune system. And when it comes to optimizing your health, incorporating superfoods into your raw food diet can take your wellness journey to the next level.

Superfoods are nutrient-rich foods that are exceptionally beneficial for our health due to their high content of vitamins, minerals, antioxidants, and phytochemicals. These powerhouse foods can help protect against chronic diseases, boost our immune system, and enhance overall vitality. Whether you follow a raw vegan, raw paleo, raw fruitarian, raw juice, raw vegetarian, raw dairy-free, raw gluten-free, raw nut-based, raw alkaline, or raw superfood diet, there are superfoods that can complement your chosen dietary path.

One of the most popular superfoods for health-conscious individuals is kale. This leafy green is packed with essential nutrients such as iron, calcium, and vitamins A, C, and K. It is a versatile ingredient that can be enjoyed in salads, smoothies, or even as crispy kale chips. Another superfood that is often incorporated into raw food diets is chia seeds. These tiny seeds are a fantastic source of omega-3 fatty acids, fiber, and protein. They can be added to your morning smoothies, sprinkled on top of salads, or used to make delicious chia puddings.
For those following a raw paleo or raw fruitarian diet, incorporating berries into your meals is an excellent choice. Berries, such as blueberries, strawberries, and raspberries, are bursting with

antioxidants and are low in sugar. They can be enjoyed as a snack, added to smoothies, or used as toppings for raw desserts.

If you are a fan of raw juices, consider adding wheatgrass or spirulina to your blends. These superfoods are rich in chlorophyll, which supports detoxification and boosts energy levels. They can easily be incorporated into your daily juice routine for an added health kick.

Regardless of your chosen raw food diet, incorporating superfoods can greatly enhance your overall health and well-being. Remember to listen to your body and experiment with different superfoods to find the ones that work best for you. By embracing a raw food lifestyle and incorporating superfoods, you are taking a significant step towards achieving optimal health and vitality.

Tips for Sustaining a Raw Food Lifestyle

Living a raw food lifestyle can be incredibly beneficial for your health and overall well-being. Whether you follow a raw food diet, raw vegan diet, raw paleo diet, raw fruitarian diet, raw juice diet, raw vegetarian diet, raw dairy-free diet, raw gluten-free diet, raw nut-based diet, raw alkaline diet, or raw superfood diet, these tips will help you sustain your chosen lifestyle and maximize its benefits.

1. Embrace variety: Incorporating a wide range of fruits, vegetables, nuts, seeds, and superfoods into your diet ensures that you receive a broad spectrum of nutrients. Experiment with different flavors, textures, and colors to keep your meals interesting and enjoyable.

2. Plan your meals: Meal planning is essential for maintaining a raw food lifestyle. Take the time to prepare your meals in advance, ensuring that you have access to fresh, nutritious options throughout the day. This will prevent you from reaching for processed or unhealthy alternatives when hunger strikes.

3. Stay hydrated: Drinking enough water is vital for overall health, and especially important when following a raw food lifestyle. Hydration helps flush out toxins, supports digestion, and aids in nutrient absorption. Make sure to drink plenty of water throughout the day, and consider incorporating hydrating fruits and vegetables into your meals.

4. Listen to your body: Pay attention to how certain foods make you feel. Each individual is

unique, and what works for one person may not work for another. Notice how your body reacts to different raw foods and adjust your diet accordingly. This will help you identify any sensitivities or allergies and allow you to make informed choices about what to include or avoid.

5. Stay connected: Surround yourself with like-minded individuals who share your passion for a raw food lifestyle. Join raw food communities, attend workshops, or connect with others through social media platforms. Having a support system can provide motivation, inspiration, and a sense of belonging.

6. Practice mindful eating: Take the time to fully experience your meals by eating slowly, savoring each bite, and paying attention to the flavors and textures. This will not only enhance your enjoyment of food but also promote better digestion and nutrient absorption.

7. Get creative in the kitchen: Experiment with different raw food recipes and techniques to keep your meals exciting and diverse. Explore new flavors, textures, and combinations to prevent boredom and ensure you receive a wide range of nutrients.

Remember, sustaining a raw food lifestyle is a journey, not a destination. Be patient with yourself, allow room for flexibility, and focus on progress rather than perfection. By incorporating these tips into your daily routine, you will be well on your way to reaping the countless benefits of a raw food lifestyle.

Overcoming Challenges and Staying Motivated

In the journey towards adopting a raw food lifestyle, challenges are bound to arise. Whether you are following a raw vegan, raw paleo, raw fruitarian, raw juice, raw vegetarian, raw dairy-free, raw gluten-free, raw nut-based, raw alkaline, or raw superfood diet, it's essential to have strategies in place to overcome these obstacles and stay motivated. This subchapter will provide you with valuable insights and practical tips to help you navigate through these challenges, ensuring your success on the path to optimal health.

One common challenge faced by health-conscious individuals is the lack of variety in raw food options. It can be easy to fall into a monotonous routine, especially when you are limited to certain food groups. To overcome this, it's important to explore new recipes, experiment with different combinations, and embrace the abundance of raw fruits, vegetables, nuts, and seeds available. By incorporating a wide variety of ingredients into your meals, you'll not only enhance the nutritional profile but also keep your taste buds satisfied.

Another challenge is the social aspect of eating raw. Dining out or attending social gatherings can be tricky when the majority of people around you are not following a raw food lifestyle. However, with a little planning and communication, you can overcome this hurdle. Research raw-friendly restaurants in your area and suggest these options when dining with friends or family. Alternatively, offer to bring a raw dish to potlucks or gatherings, showcasing the delicious and vibrant flavors of raw cuisine. By taking proactive steps, you can ensure that social events don't derail your commitment to a raw food diet.

Staying motivated is key on this journey, especially when faced with temptations or when the results aren't immediate. One strategy to stay motivated is to set realistic goals and celebrate small victories along the way. Remember that adopting a raw food lifestyle is a long-term commitment to your health and well-being. Surround yourself with like-minded individuals, join online communities, and seek out support from others who share your passion for raw food. By connecting with others who are on a similar path, you'll find encouragement, inspiration, and a sense of belonging.

Overcoming challenges and staying motivated on a raw food diet requires determination, creativity, and a supportive community. By embracing variety in your meals, finding raw-friendly options when dining out, and setting realistic goals, you can successfully navigate the obstacles that come your way. Remember, the raw food revolution is not just a dietary choice; it's a lifestyle that promotes vibrant health, increased energy, and overall well-being. Stay motivated, believe in yourself, and enjoy the incredible benefits that a raw food diet can offer.

Creating a Personalized Raw Food Plan

In today's health-conscious world, there are various diets that have gained popularity for their potential health benefits. One such diet is the raw food diet, which involves consuming unprocessed, uncooked, and mostly organic foods. Whether you follow a raw vegan, raw paleo, raw fruitarian, raw juice, raw vegetarian, raw dairy-free, raw gluten-free, raw nut-based, raw alkaline, or raw superfood diet, creating a personalized raw food plan is essential to ensure optimal health and well-being.

The first step in creating a personalized raw food plan is to understand your specific dietary needs and preferences. This can be determined by considering your individual goals, such as weight loss, improved digestion, increased energy levels, or overall well-being. Assessing your current health status and any existing health conditions is also crucial in tailoring a plan that meets your unique requirements.

Once you have identified your goals and assessed your health status, it is important to research and understand the principles and guidelines of your chosen raw food diet niche. Each niche has its own set of rules regarding the types of foods that can be consumed and the proportions in which they should be consumed. For example, a raw vegan diet excludes all animal products, while a raw paleo diet permits the consumption of raw animal products.

Next, consider your lifestyle and availability of raw food options in your area. Determine the feasibility of sourcing fresh, organic, and raw ingredients that align with your chosen diet. If certain foods are not readily available, explore alternative options or consider incorporating supplements to ensure you are meeting all your nutritional needs.

Variety is key when creating a personalized raw food plan. Aim to include a wide range of fruits, vegetables, nuts, seeds, and sprouted grains in your diet. Experiment with different flavors, textures, and preparation methods to keep your meals interesting and enjoyable.

To ensure you are obtaining all the necessary nutrients, it may be beneficial to consult with a registered dietitian or nutritionist who specializes in raw food diets. They can provide expert advice and guidance tailored to your specific needs and help you create a well-balanced and nourishing raw food plan.

Lastly, monitor your progress and make adjustments as needed. Keep track of how your body responds to the raw food plan and make any necessary modifications to optimize your health and well-being.

Creating a personalized raw food plan requires careful consideration of your individual goals, dietary preferences, and health status. By tailoring your raw food plan to meet your unique needs, you can embark on a journey towards improved health and vitality.

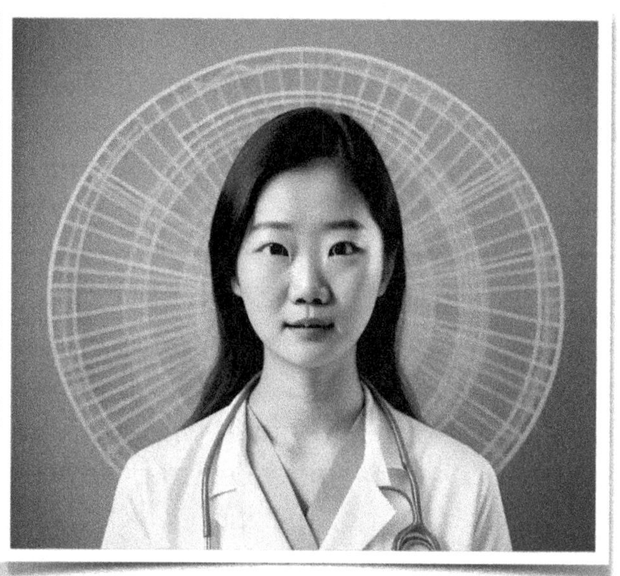

Chapter 15: Frequently Asked Questions about Raw Food Diets

Addressing Common Concerns and Misconceptions

In the world of health and nutrition, there are numerous diets and lifestyles to choose from. For health-conscious individuals, the raw food diet has gained significant popularity in recent years.

However, with any new approach to eating, there are bound to be concerns and misconceptions. In this subchapter, we aim to address some of the most common ones and shed light on the truth behind them.

One of the main concerns people have when considering a raw food diet is whether they will get enough nutrients. It is a common misconception that a raw food diet lacks essential vitamins and minerals. However, when properly planned, a raw food diet can provide all the necessary nutrients for optimal health. By incorporating a variety of fruits, vegetables, nuts, seeds, and sprouts, one can obtain a well-rounded nutrient profile.

Another concern often raised is the risk of foodborne illnesses. While it is true that certain foods, such as raw meat and dairy, can pose a higher risk, a raw food diet focuses on plant-based foods that are typically safer to consume raw. Additionally, proper food handling and hygiene practices can minimize the risk of contamination.

Some individuals worry about the lack of protein in a raw food diet. However, plant-based foods like nuts, seeds, legumes, and leafy greens are excellent sources of protein. By combining different sources and ensuring sufficient calorie intake, meeting protein requirements is easily achievable.

A common misconception is that a raw food diet is restrictive and boring. On the contrary, the raw food world offers a vast array of delicious and creative options. From raw vegan pizzas to decadent desserts made from fruits and nuts, the possibilities are endless. Exploring recipes and experimenting with different flavors can make the raw food journey exciting and satisfying.

Lastly, some people wonder if a raw food diet is sustainable in the long term. While it may not be suitable for everyone, many individuals have successfully maintained a raw food lifestyle for years, even decades. It all comes down to personal preference, commitment, and proper planning to ensure a balanced diet.

In conclusion, addressing common concerns and misconceptions surrounding the raw food diet is crucial for health-conscious individuals considering this lifestyle. By dispelling myths and providing accurate information, we hope to empower readers to make informed choices and embark on a raw food journey with confidence. Remember, knowledge is key, and with the right approach, the raw food revolution can unlock a world of vibrant health and wellness.

Troubleshooting Common Issues

As health conscious individuals, we understand the importance of nourishing our bodies with wholesome, natural foods. The raw food revolution has taken the world by storm, with various diets such as raw vegan, raw paleo, raw fruitarian, and more, gaining popularity. However, embarking on a raw food journey may come with its own set of challenges. In this subchapter, we will discuss some common issues that you may encounter and provide effective troubleshooting solutions to help you stay on track.

One common issue that raw food enthusiasts often face is a lack of variety in their meals. While raw fruits and vegetables form the foundation of a raw food diet, it's essential to incorporate a diverse range of ingredients to ensure you receive all the necessary nutrients. Experiment with different types of fruits, vegetables, nuts, seeds, and superfoods to add excitement to your meals. Consider joining raw food communities or attending workshops to learn new recipes and techniques.

Another issue that can arise is the temptation to indulge in processed or cooked foods, especially when dining out or attending social events. It's crucial to plan ahead and be prepared for such situations. Carry raw snacks or a pre-made meal with you, so you're never caught off guard. Additionally, communicate your dietary preferences to friends and family, so they can accommodate your needs during gatherings.

Digestive issues are not uncommon when transitioning to a raw food diet. The sudden increase in fiber intake can lead to bloating, gas, or irregular bowel movements. To alleviate these issues, start by introducing raw foods gradually into your diet and ensure you're properly hydrating. Chew your food thoroughly to aid digestion and consider incorporating fermented foods, such as sauerkraut or kefir, to promote a healthy gut.

Maintaining a balanced raw food diet that meets all your nutritional needs can be a challenge. It's important to educate yourself about the essential nutrients your body requires and ensure you're obtaining them from various sources. If you're concerned about specific nutrients, consider consulting with a registered dietitian who specializes in raw food diets.

While the raw food diet offers numerous health benefits, it may not be suitable for everyone. If you're experiencing prolonged feelings of fatigue, weakness, or any adverse symptoms, it's crucial to consult with a healthcare professional to rule out any underlying health conditions.

By addressing these common issues and providing troubleshooting solutions, this subchapter aims to empower health-conscious individuals following raw food diets. Remember, with a little knowledge and preparation, you can overcome these challenges and experience the full benefits of the raw food revolution.

Expert Answers and InsightsWhether you follow a raw vegan, raw paleo, raw fruitarian, raw juice, raw vegetarian, raw dairy-free, raw gluten-free, raw nut-based, raw alkaline, or raw superfood diet, this chapter is designed to provide valuable information to support your health journey.

Our team of experts, including nutritionists, dieticians, and experienced practitioners of raw food diets, have come together to answer some of the most frequently asked questions in each niche. From the benefits of a raw food diet to tips for maintaining a balanced nutrient intake, we cover a wide range of topics to help you make informed decisions about your dietary choices.

Discover the science behind raw food diets, including the impact of cooking on nutrient content and the potential benefits of consuming foods in their natural state. Our experts share their insights on the potential health advantages of raw food diets, such as increased energy levels, improved digestion, and enhanced nutrient absorption.

We also address common concerns related to specific niches within the raw food diet community. Are raw vegan diets nutritionally adequate? How can you ensure you're getting enough protein on a raw paleo diet? What are the best sources of vitamins and minerals for raw fruitarians? These are just a few of the questions our experts answer, providing clarity and guidance for those following niche raw food diets.

Additionally, we explore the practical aspects of raw food diets, offering tips and tricks for meal planning, food preparation, and dining out. Our experts provide advice on sourcing high-quality raw ingredients, kitchen equipment essentials, and creative recipes to keep your raw food journey exciting and diverse.

Whether you're a seasoned practitioner or just starting out on a raw food diet, "Expert Answers and Insights" is a valuable resource that will empower you to make informed decisions about your health and nutrition. Get ready to unlock the full potential of raw food diets and embark on a journey towards optimal well-being.

Remember, always consult with a qualified healthcare professional before making any significant changes to your diet or lifestyle.

Chapter 16: Conclusion

Embracing the Raw Food Revolution

In recent years, there has been a growing movement towards embracing a raw food lifestyle. This revolutionary approach to eating focuses on consuming unprocessed, uncooked, and plant-based foods in their natural state. Welcome to the world of the raw food revolution!

For health-conscious individuals seeking to improve their well-being, the raw food revolution offers an exciting and transformative way of nourishing the body. Whether you follow a raw food diet, raw vegan diet, raw paleo diet, raw fruitarian diet, raw juice diet, raw vegetarian diet, raw dairy-free diet, raw gluten-free diet, raw nut-based diet, raw alkaline diet, or raw superfood diet, this subchapter has something to offer you.

Raw food diets are centered around the principle that cooking destroys essential nutrients and enzymes present in food. By consuming raw foods, individuals can benefit from higher nutrient absorption, improved digestion, increased energy levels, and a stronger immune system. The raw food revolution encourages individuals to fill their plates with a colorful array of fruits, vegetables, nuts, seeds, and sprouted grains.

If you are a raw vegan enthusiast, the raw food revolution provides an abundance of plant-based options to fuel your body. From nutrient-packed smoothies and juices to vibrant salads and delectable raw desserts, the possibilities are endless. Discover the joy of experimenting with unique ingredients and creating delicious meals that are not only good for your health but also good for the planet.

Are you a raw paleo adherent? The raw food revolution has got you covered too! Explore the wealth of raw, unprocessed, and organic animal products such as raw dairy, eggs, and fermented foods to support your primal lifestyle. Embrace the simplicity of eating foods that our ancestors thrived on, while reaping the benefits of improved digestion, increased vitality, and enhanced mental clarity.

No matter your specific dietary niche within the raw food revolution, one thing is certain - this lifestyle is a gateway to optimal health and well-being. So, join the movement and embrace the raw food revolution today. Discover a world filled with vibrant flavors, nourishing meals, and a renewed sense of vitality. It's time to unlock the potential of your health through the power of raw food!

Final Thoughts and Encouragement for Health Conscious Individuals

Congratulations, health-conscious individuals, on embarking on the incredible journey of the raw food revolution! You have taken a significant step towards transforming your health and well-being. As you continue to explore the various niches within the raw food movement, such as raw vegan, raw paleo, raw fruitarian, raw juice, raw vegetarian, raw dairy-free, raw gluten-free, raw nut-based, raw alkaline, and raw superfood diets, we would like to offer some final thoughts and encouragement to support your ongoing commitment to a health-conscious lifestyle.

First and foremost, we want to applaud you for choosing a path that prioritizes your health and wellness. By opting for a raw food diet, you are nourishing your body with the most natural, unprocessed, and nutrient-dense foods available. This conscious decision not only benefits your physical health but also contributes to a sustainable and eco-friendly lifestyle.

As you embark on this journey, it is essential to approach it with an open mind and a willingness to experiment. Raw food diets offer a vast array of options, and it is crucial to explore the different niches to find what works best for you. Discover the foods that you enjoy and that make you feel vibrant and energized. Remember, there is no one-size-fits-all approach to the raw food revolution. Embrace the diversity and tailor your diet to suit your individual needs and preferences.

It is also important to stay informed and educated about the raw food movement. Continuously seek out reliable sources of information, books, blogs, and documentaries that can deepen your understanding of the benefits and potential challenges of a raw food diet. Knowledge empowers you to make informed decisions and adapt your lifestyle as needed.

While embarking on any new dietary journey, it is crucial to practice self-compassion and patience. Rome wasn't built in a day, and transitioning to a raw food diet takes time and effort. There may be moments when you face challenges or setbacks, but remember that every step forward counts. Surround yourself with a supportive community of like-minded individuals who can provide guidance, motivation, and encouragement along the way.

Lastly, never forget to celebrate your successes, no matter how small they may seem. Each day that you choose to prioritize your health and nourish your body with raw, wholesome foods is a victory worth acknowledging. Embrace the incredible potential of the raw food revolution to transform your health, enhance your vitality, and create a positive impact on the world around you.

In conclusion, congratulations to all you health-conscious individuals for pursuing a raw food diet. Your commitment to a healthier lifestyle and the exploration of various niches within the raw food movement is commendable. As you continue on this path, remember to stay open-minded, informed, patient, and compassionate towards yourself. Celebrate your journey, and embrace the incredible potential of the raw food revolution to revolutionize your health and well-being.

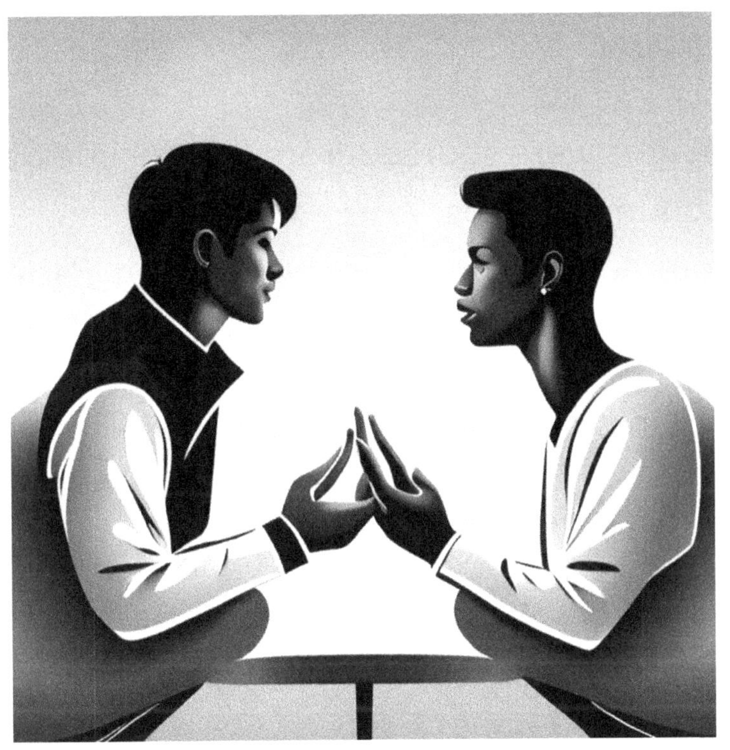

WAR OF IDEAS

warofideas.shop

Images were sourced from the Wikimedia Commons, https://commons.wikimedia.org/wiki/Main_Page

This files are licensed under the Creative Commons Attribution 2.0 Generic license.

Also images were created with imagine.art/ai

Special Thanks to: Greg Schlegel, Joshua Davenport.

Research assisted through Claude AI, created by Anthropic, which is an AI safety and research company. They build reliable, interpretable, and steerable AI systems. https://www.anthropic.com/company

About the Author

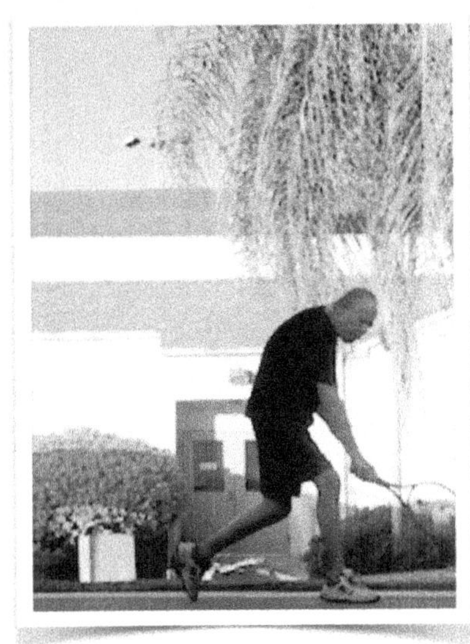

William Davenport (born 1960, Evansville, Indiana) is a filmmaker, musician, publisher, writer, teacher and political activist. He is best known for his films about autism, music and politics, also for his work as the publisher of Unsound magazine, and as the founding member of the experimental band Problemist.